B. SAVAGE

Calisthenics for Beginners

Contents

1 The Basics — 1

2 Optional Equipment — 5

3 Week 1: Building Foundations — 7

4 Monday — 8

5 Tuesday — 11

6 Wednesday — 13

7 Thursday — 15

8 Friday — 16

9 Saturday — 18

10 Sunday — 19

11 Week 1: Progress Tracker — 20

12 Week 2: Building Strength and Stamina — 22

13 Monday — 23

14 Tuesday — 25

15 Wednesday — 27

16 Thursday — 29

17 Friday — 30

18 Saturday — 32

19 Sunday — 33

20 Week 2: Progress Tracker — 34

21 Week 3: Strengthening Foundations — 36

22 Monday — 37

23 Tuesday — 39

24 Wednesday — 41

25 Thursday — 43

26 Friday   44

27 Saturday   46

28 Sunday   47

29 Week 3: Progress Tracker   48

30 Week 4: Mastering Foundations   50

31 Monday   51

32 Tuesday   53

33 Wednesday   55

34 Thursday   57

35 Friday   58

36 Saturday   60

37 Sunday   61

38 Week 4: Progress Tracker   62

39 You Did It!   64

40 GLOSSARY   65

1

The Basics

THE BASICS:

4-Week Beginner Calisthenics Training Program

Duration: 4 Weeks

Welcome to "THE BASICS," a 4-week beginner's journey into the world of calisthenics. This program is thoughtfully designed to introduce you to foundational techniques and help you build a strong base for your calisthenics journey. Our primary focus is on enhancing your strength, flexibility, and body control through progressive exercises. Over these 4 weeks, you'll develop a solid foundation, setting the stage for future programs in this series.

Overview:

In these 4 weeks, your goal is to give it your all and complete each day's workout to the best of your ability. At the beginning, you might not be able to finish every exercise, but that's okay! With dedication and consistency, you'll see significant improvements. Feel free to modify the workouts and use assistance bands as needed to maintain proper form. Once you complete this 4-week program, you'll be prepared to dive into intermediate calisthenic skills on your way to mastering some of the most impressive advanced calisthenic movements. Let's get started!

The Weekly Progress Check is a tool to help individuals gauge their readiness to transition from beginner to intermediate calisthenics training. It assesses your strength and skill levels in key exercises. Here's a general summary of how to interpret the results:

Pull-Ups:

- 0-3 reps: You're in the early stages of pull-up development. Focus on increasing your pull-up strength before progressing.
- 4-6 reps: You're making progress, but there's room for improvement. Continue building strength with pull-ups.
- 7-9 reps: Your pull-up strength is approaching an intermediate level. Consider moving to intermediate training when you consistently reach 7 or more reps.
- 10+ reps: You have achieved an intermediate level of pull-up strength. You're ready for more challenging exercises in intermediate training.

Dips:

- 0-3 reps: Begin by building your dip strength. Aim for at least 4-6 reps before transitioning to intermediate training.
- 4-6 reps: You're on the right track, but you can improve further. Strive for 7-9 reps for a smoother transition.
- 7-9 reps: Your dip strength is approaching an intermediate level.

When you consistently hit 7 or more reps, consider moving forward.

- 10+ reps: You've attained an intermediate level of dip strength. You're ready for more advanced exercises in intermediate training.

L-Sit Hold:

- <10 seconds: Work on improving your core strength and balance. Aim for 10-20 seconds before transitioning.
- 10-20 seconds: You're progressing well. Continue to extend your hold time. Aim for 21-30 seconds to move on.
- 21-30 seconds: Your L-sit hold is getting strong. When you consistently reach >30 seconds, consider the next level.
- 30 seconds: You've developed an intermediate level L-sit hold. You're ready to tackle more advanced core exercises.

Wall Handstand Push-Ups:

- 0-2 reps: Start by improving your upper body and shoulder strength. Aim for 3-5 reps for an intermediate readiness.
- 3-5 reps: You're making progress. Continue to work on your wall handstand push-ups. Aim for 6-8 reps for a transition.
- 6-8 reps: Your shoulder strength is improving. Consistently hitting 9+ reps signals readiness for intermediate training.
- 9+ reps: You've achieved an intermediate level of shoulder strength. You can now explore more advanced exercises.

One-Arm Push-Up Progressions:

- 0-1 rep: Begin by mastering regular push-ups. Progress to 2-3 reps before attempting one-arm push-up progressions.
- 2-3 reps: You're getting there. Work on your one-arm push-up

progressions, aiming for 4-5 reps to advance.

- 4-5 reps: Your one-arm push-up progressions are improving. Consistently hitting 6 or more reps means you're ready for intermediates.
- 6+ reps: You've reached an intermediate level with one-arm push-up progressions. Transition to more advanced training.

Chest to Bar Pull-Ups:

- 0-2 reps: Start with regular pull-ups and focus on reaching chest-to-bar height. Aim for 3-4 reps for intermediate readiness.
- 3-4 reps: You're on the right track. Keep working on chest-to-bar pull-ups, aiming for 5-6 reps to move forward.
- 5-6 reps: Your chest-to-bar pull-ups are improving. When you consistently reach 7 or more reps, consider intermediate training.
- 7+ reps: You've attained an intermediate level with chest-to-bar pull-ups. You're ready for more challenging workouts.

Remember that these guidelines are approximate and individual progress may vary. It's essential to maintain proper form, avoid over training, and listen to your body throughout your calisthenics journey. Consistency, patience, and dedication will help you reach your calisthenics goals.

2

Optional Equipment

- Exercise Mat: An exercise mat is essential for providing a comfortable surface for various exercises, especially floor-based movements like push-ups, planks, and core exercises.
- Resistance Bands: You'll need resistance bands for assistance in exercises like assisted pull-ups, band-assisted pistol squats, and other resistance-based movements.
- Pull-Up Bar: A pull-up bar is required for practicing pull-ups, hanging leg raises, and other exercises that involve gripping a bar.
- Jump Rope: A jump rope is used for warm-up and cardio exercises to improve endurance and coordination.
- Medicine Ball (optional): Though optional, a medicine ball can be used for exercises like medicine ball slams to add extra resistance and variety to your workouts.
- Bench or Stable Chair: You'll need a bench or stable chair for dips and incline push-ups.
- Yoga Mat (optional): If you plan to incorporate yoga or stretching routines into your active rest days, a yoga mat can be helpful.
- Foam Roller: A foam roller is used for foam rolling, which aids in

muscle recovery and mobility.
- Comfortable Workout Clothing: Wear comfortable workout attire and proper athletic shoes to ensure safety and comfort during your workouts.
- Water Bottle: Staying hydrated is crucial during exercise, so have a water bottle handy.
- Timer or Stopwatch: You'll need a timer or stopwatch to keep track of rest intervals and exercise duration.
- Reflective and Rest Day Materials: On your rest and reflection days, you'll need materials for reflection, setting goals, and planning the upcoming week's workouts.

Please note that the specifics of equipment may vary based on your preferences and what you have available. Additionally, as you progress in your calisthenics journey, you might invest in additional equipment to meet your evolving needs and goals. Always prioritize safety, proper form, and gradual progression throughout the program.

3

Week 1: Building Foundations

Duration: 7 days

Weekly Schedule:

- Monday: Legs and Abs
- Tuesday: Push Day
- Wednesday: Pull Day
- Thursday: Active Rest Day
- Friday: Full Body
- Saturday: Active Rest Day
- Sunday: Rest

4

Monday

Legs and Abs - Laying the Groundwork
Overview:

Welcome to Week 1 of your calisthenics journey! This week, we're focusing on building the foundational strength and skills you'll need to progress in calisthenics. Today, it's all about your lower body and core. We'll be working towards mastering unassisted pistol squats, an essential calisthenic skill.

Progression Path:

- Beginner: Body weight squats
- Advanced Beginner: Assisted single-leg squats
- Advanced: Eccentric pistol squats
- Elite Beginner: Full pistol squats

Warm-Up (10-15 minutes):

- Jog in place: 3 minutes

- Leg swings: 10 reps each leg
- Arm circles: 10 reps each arm
- Hip circles: 10 reps each direction

Legs and Abs Workout:

- Pistol Squat Progressions - Goal: unassisted pistol squats
- Body weight Squats: 2 sets x 15 reps
- Assisted Single-Leg Squats: 2 sets x 8 reps each leg
- Eccentric Pistol Squats: 2 sets x 5 reps each leg
- Full Pistol Squats (when ready): Aim for 10 reps each leg

Superset Cycles (Repeat 2x):

Cycle 1:

- Split Squats: 1 set x 10 reps per leg
- Side lunges (Hack Squat): 1 set x 10 reps per leg
- Lunges (Alternating Legs): 1 set x 12 reps per leg
- Russian Twists: 1 set x 15 reps per side

Cycle 2:

- Explosive Split Squats: 1 set x 10 reps per leg
- Jump Squats: 1 set x 15 reps
- L-Sit (advanced hanging L-Sit) Leg Raises: 1 set x 10-12 reps

Finisher Exercises:

- Calf Raises: 3 sets x 15 reps
- Glute Bridges: 3 sets x 15 reps

- Finisher Circuit (Repeat 2x):
- Jumping Lunges: 30 seconds
- Bicycle Crunches: 30 seconds
- Plank: Hold for maximum time

5

Tuesday

Push Day - Building Upper Body Strength
  Overview:

Day 2 is all about building upper body strength and progressing towards advanced push-up variations. By mastering these basics, you'll lay the groundwork for advanced beginner calisthenic skills in the future.

Progression Path:

- Beginner: Regular push-ups
- Advanced Beginner: Diamond push-ups
- Advanced: Beast pose to push-up to squat
- Elite Beginner: Tiger bend push-ups

Warm-Up (10-15 minutes):

- Jump rope: 3 minutes
- Push-up to Downward Dog: 10 reps
- Chest openers: 10 reps each side

- Wrist stretches: 1 minute

Push Day Workout:

- Regular Push-Ups: 3 sets of 10 reps
- Diamond Push-Ups: 3 sets x 8-12 reps
- Beast Pose to Push-Up to Squat: 3 sets of 10 reps
- Tiger Bend Push-Ups: Perform 3 sets of 2-10 reps (gradually increasing difficulty)
- Dips: 3 sets x 8-12 reps (band assistance if needed)
- Beginner Band overhead press: Progress to heavier bands
- Handstand Practice Against Wall: 3 sets x 30-60 seconds
- Pike Push-Ups: 3 sets x 8-10 reps

Finisher Circuit (Repeat 2x):

- Push-Up Variations: 30 seconds
- Tricep Dips: 30 seconds
- Burpees: 30 seconds
- Superman Planks: 30 seconds

6

Wednesday

Pull Day - Building Upper Body and Core Strength

Overview:

Welcome to Day 3, where we'll focus on building upper body and core strength. These exercises are your stepping stones to pull-up mastery, one of the advanced beginner calisthenic skills we'll be working towards.

Progression Path:

- Beginner: Band-assisted pull-ups
- Advanced Beginner: Hanging L-sit holds
- Advanced: Band-assisted pistol squats
- Elite Beginner: Unassisted pull-ups

Warm-Up (10-15 minutes):

- Arm swings: 10 reps each arm
- Band pull-aparts: 15 reps
- Scapular shrugs: 10 reps

- Jumping jacks: 30 seconds

Pull Day Workout:

Superset Cycles (Repeat 2x):

Cycle 1:

- Band Assisted Pull-Ups: 1 set x 6-10 reps
- Hanging L-Sit Holds: 1 set (for time or max effort)
- Band or Chair Assisted Pistol Squats: 1 set x 3 reps each leg

Cycle 2:

- Band Assisted Pull-Ups: 1 set x 6-10 reps
- Hanging Knees to Elbows: 1 set (1-10 reps) do progressions
- Band or Chair Assisted Pistol Squats: 1 set x 3 reps each leg

Finisher Exercises:

- Band Assisted High Pulls: 3 sets x 8-12 reps
- Inverted Rows: 3 sets x 10-12 reps
- Scapular Pull-Ups: 3 sets x 8-10 reps
- body weight Bicep Curls: 3 sets x 12-15 reps

Finisher Circuit (Repeat 2x):

- Pull-Ups or Chin-Ups: 30 seconds
- Plank: Hold for maximum time
- Bicycle Crunches: 30 seconds
- Russian Twists: 30 seconds

7

Thursday

Active Rest Day – Recovery and Maintenance

Overview:

Welcome to Day 4, today is your active rest day. It's essential for recovery and maintenance. Use this time to rejuvenate and prepare for upcoming workouts. Proper recovery now will pay off when you're aiming for advanced beginner calisthenic skills in the future.

Exercises:

- Light Jog or Walk: 30 minutes
- Dynamic Stretching: 15 minutes
- Foam Rolling: 10 minutes

8

Friday

Full Body – Integrating Movements
Overview:

Day 5 integrates the movements you've been working on so far. By combining these exercises, you'll build a holistic foundation for more advanced calisthenic skills in the advanced beginner category.

Progression Path:

- Beginner to Elite: Progression towards mastering each exercise

Warm-Up (10-15 minutes):

- High knees: 3 minutes
- Squat to stand: 10 reps
- Dynamic lunges: 10 reps each leg
- Shoulder circles: 10 reps each direction

Full Body Main Workout:

- Burpees: 3 sets x 12-15 reps
- Pull-Ups (Standard or Wide Grip): 3 sets x 6-8 reps
- Pistol Squat Progressions: 3 sets x 6 reps per leg
- Push-Ups (Variations): 3 sets x 10-15 reps
- L-Sit Progressions: 3 sets x 10-15 seconds

Finisher Circuit (Repeat 2x):

- Medicine Ball Slams: 30 seconds
- Kickthroughs: 30 seconds
- Mountain Climbers: 30 seconds
- Hollow Body Hold: 30 seconds
- Plank Shoulder Taps: 30 seconds

9

Saturday

Active Rest Day - Flexibility and Cardio
  Overview:

Day 6 is dedicated to active rest, focusing on flexibility and cardiovascular fitness. These elements are essential for balanced calisthenics training and future advanced beginner skills.

Progression Path:

- Active rest, no specific progression path

Exercises:

- Yoga or Light Stretching: 30 minutes
- Skipping Rope: 15 minutes

10

Sunday

Sunday: Rest - Recovery and Reflection

Overview:

On Day 7, it's time for complete rest. Allow your body and mind to recover fully, and reflect on the progress you've made this week. You're on your way to becoming an advanced beginner in the world of calisthenics!

11

Week 1: Progress Tracker

Please mark your progress for each exercise category. Aim to progress gradually from one category to the next. Consistency in training will lead to noticeable improvements.

Pull-Ups:

- [ ] 0-3
- [ ] 4-6
- [ ] 7-9
- [ ] 10+

Dips:

- [ ] 0-3
- [ ] 4-6
- [ ] 7-9
- [ ] 10+

L-Sit Hold:

- [ ] <10 seconds
- [ ] 10-20 seconds
- [ ] 21-30 seconds
- [ ] >30 seconds

Wall Handstand Push-Ups:

- [ ] 0-2
- [ ] 3-5
- [ ] 6-8
- [ ] 9+

One-Arm Push-Up Progressions:

- [ ] 0-1
- [ ] 2-3
- [ ] 4-5
- [ ] 6+

Chest to Bar Pull-Ups:

- [ ] 0-2
- [ ] 3-4
- [ ] 5-6
- [ ] 7+

12

Week 2: Building Strength and Stamina

Duration: 7 days
Weekly Schedule

- Monday: Legs and Abs
- Tuesday: Push Day
- Wednesday: Pull Day
- Thursday: Active Rest Day
- Friday: Full Body
- Saturday: Active Rest Day
- Sunday: Rest

13

Monday

Legs and Abs - Building Lower Body Power

Overview:

Welcome to Week 2! We're continuing to build strength and stamina. Today, we're focusing on lower body power and core stability.

Progression Path:

- Beginner: Body weight squats
- Advanced Beginner: Assisted pistol squats with bands
- Advanced: Full pistol squats
- Elite Beginner: Bulgarian split squats

Warm-Up (10-15 minutes):

- Jog in place: 3 minutes
- Leg swings: 10 reps each leg
- Arm circles: 10 reps each arm
- Hip circles: 10 reps each direction

Legs and Abs Workout:

- Bulgarian Split Squats: 3 sets x 10 reps per leg
- Reverse Lunges: 3 sets x 12 reps per leg
- Leg Raises: 3 sets x 15 reps
- Plank: 3 sets x 30-45 seconds

Superset Cycles (Repeat 2x):

Cycle 1:

- Body weight Squats: 2 sets x 15 reps
- Russian Twists: 2 sets x 15 reps per side

Cycle 2:

- Jump Squats: 2 sets x 12 reps
- L-Sit (on the floor) Leg Raises: 2 sets x 10-12 reps

Finisher Circuit (Repeat 2x):

- Box Jumps (if available): 1 set x 10 reps
- Bicycle Crunches: 1 set x 20 reps per side
- Standing Calf Raises: 1 set x 20 reps

14

Tuesday

Push Day - Upper Body Endurance
Overview:

Day 2 is all about building upper body endurance and preparing for advanced push-up variations.

Progression Path:

- Beginner: Push-ups with knees on the floor
- Advanced Beginner: Regular push-ups
- Advanced: Diamond push-ups
- Elite Beginner: Wide push-ups

Warm-Up (10-15 minutes):

- Jump rope: 3 minutes
- Push-up to Downward Dog: 10 reps
- Chest openers: 10 reps each side
- Wrist stretches: 1 minute

Push Day Workout:

- Regular Push-Ups: 3 sets x 12-15 reps
- Diamond Push-Ups: 3 sets x 10-12 reps
- Wide Push-Ups: 3 sets x 12-15 reps
- Incline Push-Ups (hands on a bench or step): 3 sets x 15 reps
- Dips: 3 sets x 8-10 reps

Superset Cycles (Repeat 2x):

Cycle 1:

- Plank: 2 sets x 30 seconds
- Shoulder Taps: 2 sets x 15 reps per side

Cycle 2:

- Tricep Dips (use a sturdy chair or parallel bars): 2 sets x 10-12 reps
- Side Plank (each side): 2 sets x 20-30 seconds

Finisher Exercises:

- Push-Up Hold (hold at the midpoint of a push-up): 2 sets x 30 seconds
- Standing Wall Angels (with back against the wall): 2 sets x 10 reps
- Medicine Ball Chest Pass (if available): 2 sets x 15 reps

15

Wednesday

Wednesday: Pull Day - Developing Upper Body Strength
   Overview:

Welcome to Day 3. We're focusing on building upper body strength and core stability. These exercises will help you progress towards pull-up mastery.

Progression Path:

- Beginner: Band-assisted pull-ups
- Advanced Beginner: Negative pull-ups
- Advanced: Pull-ups with resistance bands
- Elite Beginner: Unassisted pull-ups

Warm-Up (10-15 minutes):

- Arm swings: 10 reps each arm
- Band pull-aparts: 15 reps
- Scapular shrugs: 10 reps

- Jumping jacks: 30 seconds

Pull Day Workout:

- Pull-Ups (Assisted or Unassisted): 3 sets x 6-8 reps
- Negative Pull-Ups (lowering yourself slowly): 3 sets x 3-5 reps
- Band Face Pulls: 3 sets x 12-15 reps
- Hanging Leg Raises: 3 sets x 10-12 reps
- Bent Over Rows (use a broomstick or light object): 3 sets x 12 reps
- Superset Cycles (Repeat 2x):

Cycle 1:

- Band Pull-Aparts: 2 sets x 15 reps
- Bicep Curls (use a broomstick or light object): 2 sets x 15 reps

Cycle 2:

- Scapular Shrugs: 2 sets x 15 reps
- Hollow Body Holds: 2 sets x 20-30 seconds

Finisher Circuit (Repeat 2x):

- Jumping Pull-Ups (assisted if needed): 1 set x 12-15 reps
- Russian Twists: 1 set x 20 reps per side
- Standing Calf Raises: 1 set x 20 reps

16

Thursday

Thursday: Active Rest Day – Recovery and Mobility

Overview:

Welcome to Day 4, today is your active rest day. Focus on recovery and mobility to prepare for the remaining workouts of the week.

Active Rest Activities:

- Light Jog or Walk: 30 minutes
- Dynamic Stretching: 15 minutes
- Foam Rolling: 10 minutes

17

Friday

Friday: Full Body - Integrating Movements
  Overview:

Day 5 integrates various movements to build a holistic foundation for advanced beginner calisthenic skills.
  Progression Path:

- Beginner to Elite: Progression towards mastering each exercise

Warm-Up (10-15 minutes):

- High knees: 3 minutes
- Squat to stand: 10 reps
- Dynamic lunges: 10 reps each leg
- Shoulder circles: 10 reps each direction

Full Body Main Workout:

- Burpees: 3 sets x 12-15 reps

- Pull-Ups (Standard or Wide Grip): 3 sets x 6-8 reps
- Pistol Squat Progressions: 3 sets x 6 reps per leg
- Push-Ups (Variations): 3 sets x 10-15 reps
- L-Sit Progressions: 3 sets x 10-15 seconds
- Plank: 3 sets x 30-45 seconds

Finisher Circuit (Repeat 2x):

- Box Jumps (if available): 1 set x 10 reps
- Bicycle Crunches: 1 set x 20 reps per side
- Standing Calf Raises: 1 set x 20 reps

18

Saturday

Active Rest Day – Flexibility and Cardio
  Overview:

Day 6 focuses on flexibility and cardiovascular fitness, essential for balanced calisthenics training and future skills.

Active Rest Activities:

- Yoga or Light Stretching: 30 minutes
- Skipping Rope: 15 minutes

19

Sunday

Rest - Recovery and Reflection

Overview:

On Day 7, take complete rest. Allow your body and mind to recover fully and reflect on your progress during the week.

Rest Day Activities:

- Rest and relaxation
- Reflect on your accomplishments and set goals for the upcoming week
- Weekly Progress Check - Tracking Your Journey:

20

Week 2: Progress Tracker

Please mark your progress for each exercise category. Aim to progress gradually from one category to the next. Consistency in training will lead to noticeable improvements.

Pull-Ups:

- [ ] 0-3
- [ ] 4-6
- [ ] 7-9
- [ ] 10+

Dips:

- [ ] 0-3
- [ ] 4-6
- [ ] 7-9
- [ ] 10+

L-Sit Hold:

- [ ] <10 seconds
- [ ] 10-20 seconds
- [ ] 21-30 seconds
- [ ] >30 seconds

Wall Handstand Push-Ups:

- [ ] 0-2
- [ ] 3-5
- [ ] 6-8
- [ ] 9+

One-Arm Push-Up Progressions:

- [ ] 0-1
- [ ] 2-3
- [ ] 4-5
- [ ] 6+

Chest to Bar Pull-Ups:

- [ ] 0-2
- [ ] 3-4
- [ ] 5-6
- [ ] 7+

21

Week 3: Strengthening Foundations

Duration: 7 days
Weekly Schedule

- Monday: Legs and Abs
- Tuesday: Push Day
- Wednesday: Pull Day
- Thursday: Active Rest Day
- Friday: Full Body
- Saturday: Active Rest Day
- Sunday: Rest

22

Monday

Legs and Abs - Strengthening the Core
Overview:

Welcome to Week 3. Today's focus is on strengthening your core muscles while working on your lower body. These exercises will help you build a solid foundation for advanced beginner calisthenic skills.

Progression Path:

- Beginner: Body weight squats
- Advanced Beginner: Assisted single-leg squats
- Advanced: Eccentric pistol squats
- Elite Beginner: Full pistol squats

Warm-Up (10-15 minutes):

- Jog in place: 3 minutes
- Leg swings: 10 reps each leg
- Arm circles: 10 reps each arm

- Hip circles: 10 reps each direction

Legs and Abs Workout:

- Pistol Squat Progressions: Goal - unassisted pistol squats
- Body weight Squats: 2 sets x 15 reps
- Assisted Single-Leg Squats: 2 sets x 8 reps each leg
- Eccentric Pistol Squats: 2 sets x 5 reps each leg
- Full Pistol Squats (when ready): Aim for 10 reps each leg

Superset Cycles (Repeat 2x):

Cycle 1:

- Split Squats: 1 set x 10 reps per leg
- Side Lunges (Hack Squat): 1 set x 10 reps per leg
- Lunges (Alternating Legs): 1 set x 12 reps per leg
- Russian Twists: 1 set x 15 reps per side

Cycle 2:

- Explosive Split Squats: 1 set x 10 reps per leg
- Jump Squats: 1 set x 15 reps
- L-Sit (advanced hanging L-Sit) Leg Raises: 1 set x 10-12 reps

Finisher Exercises (Repeat 2x):

- Calf Raises: 3 sets x 15 reps
- Glute Bridges: 3 sets x 15 reps

23

Tuesday

Push Day - Advancing Upper Body Strength
  Overview:

Day 2 focuses on advancing your upper body strength through various push-up variations. These exercises are crucial for your progress in advanced beginner calisthenic skills.

Progression Path:

  - Beginner: Regular push-ups
  - Advanced Beginner: Diamond push-ups
  - Advanced: Beast pose to push-up to squat
  - Elite Beginner: Tiger bend push-ups

Warm-Up (10-15 minutes):

  - Jump rope: 3 minutes
  - Push-up to Downward Dog: 10 reps
  - Chest openers: 10 reps each side

- Wrist stretches: 1 minute

Push Day Workout:

- Regular Push-Ups: 3 sets of 10 reps
- Diamond Push-Ups: 3 sets x 8-12 reps
- Beast Pose to Push-Up to Squat: 3 sets of 10 reps
- Tiger Bend Push-Ups: Perform 3 sets of 2-10 reps (gradually increasing difficulty)
- Dips: 3 sets x 8-12 reps (band assistance if needed)
- Beginner Band overhead press: Progress to heavier bands
- Handstand Practice Against Wall: 3 sets x 30-60 seconds
- Pike Push-Ups: 3 sets x 8-10 reps

Superset Cycles (Repeat 2x):

Cycle 1:

- Plank Shoulder Taps: 30 seconds
- Jumping Jacks: 30 seconds
- Mountain Climbers: 30 seconds
- Band Shoulder Press: 30 seconds
- Burpees: 5 reps

Cycle 2:

- Band Face Pulls: 2 sets x 15 reps
- Tricep Dips (using a bench or chair): 2 sets x 10-12 reps
- Hollow Body Holds: 2 sets x 20-30 seconds

24

Wednesday

Pull Day - Developing Upper Body Strength
Overview:

Welcome to Day 3. We're focusing on building upper body strength and core stability. These exercises will help you progress towards pull-up mastery.

Progression Path:

- Beginner: Band-assisted pull-ups
- Advanced Beginner: Negative pull-ups
- Advanced: Pull-ups with resistance bands
- Elite Beginner: Unassisted pull-ups

Warm-Up (10-15 minutes):

- Arm swings: 10 reps each arm
- Band pull-aparts: 15 reps
- Scapular shrugs: 10 reps

- Jumping jacks: 30 seconds

Pull Day Workout:

- Pull-Ups (Assisted or Unassisted): 3 sets x 6-8 reps
- Negative Pull-Ups (lowering yourself slowly): 3 sets x 3-5 reps
- Band Face Pulls: 3 sets x 12-15 reps
- Hanging Leg Raises: 3 sets x 10-12 reps
- Bent Over Rows (use a broomstick or light object): 3 sets x 12 reps

Superset Cycles (Repeat 2x):

Cycle 1:

- Band Pull-Aparts: 2 sets x 15 reps
- Bicep Curls (use a broomstick or light object): 2 sets x 15 reps

Cycle 2:

- Scapular Shrugs: 2 sets x 15 reps
- Hollow Body Holds: 2 sets x 20-30 seconds

Finisher Circuit (Repeat 2x):

- Jumping Pull-Ups (assisted if needed): 1 set x 12-15 reps
- Russian Twists: 1 set x 20 reps per side
- Standing Calf Raises: 1 set x 20 reps

25

Thursday

Active Rest Day – Recovery and Mobility

Overview:

Welcome to Day 4, today is your active rest day. Focus on recovery and mobility to prepare for the remaining workouts of the week.

Active Rest Activities:

- Light Jog or Walk: 30 minutes
- Dynamic Stretching: 15 minutes
- Foam Rolling: 10 minutes

26

Friday

Full Body - Integrating Movements
  Overview:

Day 5 integrates various movements to build a holistic foundation for advanced beginner calisthenic skills.

Progression Path:

  · Beginner to Elite: Progression towards mastering each exercise

Warm-Up (10-15 minutes):

  · High knees: 3 minutes
  · Squat to stand: 10 reps
  · Dynamic lunges: 10 reps each leg
  · Shoulder circles: 10 reps each direction

Full Body Main Workout:

- Burpees: 3 sets x 12-15 reps
- Pull-Ups (Standard or Wide Grip): 3 sets x 6-8 reps
- Pistol Squat Progressions: 3 sets x 6 reps per leg
- Push-Ups (Variations): 3 sets x 10-15 reps
- L-Sit Progressions: 3 sets x 10-15 seconds
- Plank: 3 sets x 30-45 seconds

Finisher Circuit (Repeat 2x):

- Box Jumps (if available): 1 set x 10 reps
- Bicycle Crunches: 1 set x 20 reps per side
- Medicine Ball Slams (or use a heavy object): 1 set x 12 reps
- Flutter Kicks: 1 set x 30 seconds

27

Saturday

Active Rest Day – Flexibility and Cardio
Overview:

Day 6 is dedicated to active rest, focusing on flexibility and cardiovascular fitness to maintain overall balance in your calisthenics training.

Active Rest Activities:

- Yoga or Light Stretching: 30 minutes
- Skipping Rope: 15 minutes

28

Sunday

Rest – Recovery and Reflection

Overview:

On Day 7, take complete rest to allow your body and mind to recover fully. Reflect on the progress you've made throughout Week 3.

Congratulations on completing Week 3 of "THE BASICS." You're steadily progressing towards advanced beginner calisthenic skills. Keep up the consistency and proper form to continue your journey!

Week 3: Progress Tracker

Please mark your progress for each exercise category. Aim to progress gradually from one category to the next. Consistency in training will lead to noticeable improvements.

Pull-Ups:

- [ ] 0-3
- [ ] 4-6
- [ ] 7-9
- [ ] 10+

Dips:

- [ ] 0-3
- [ ] 4-6
- [ ] 7-9
- [ ] 10+

L-Sit Hold:

- [ ] <10 seconds
- [ ] 10-20 seconds
- [ ] 21-30 seconds
- [ ] >30 seconds

Wall Handstand Push-Ups:

- [ ] 0-2
- [ ] 3-5
- [ ] 6-8
- [ ] 9+

One-Arm Push-Up Progressions:

- [ ] 0-1
- [ ] 2-3
- [ ] 4-5
- [ ] 6+

Chest to Bar Pull-Ups:

- [ ] 0-2
- [ ] 3-4
- [ ] 5-6
- [ ] 7+

30

Week 4: Mastering Foundations

Duration: 7 days

Weekly Schedule

- Monday: Legs and Abs
- Tuesday: Push Day
- Wednesday: Pull Day
- Thursday: Active Rest Day
- Friday: Full Body
- Saturday: Active Rest Day
- Sunday: Rest

31

Monday

Legs and Abs - Advanced Lower Body Workout
Overview:

Welcome to Week 4, where we'll continue to challenge and refine your foundational strength and skills. Today, we focus on advanced lower body exercises to further develop your legs and core. Get ready to elevate your pistol squat game.

Progression Path:

- Beginner: Body weight squats
- Advanced Beginner: Assisted single-leg squats
- Advanced: Eccentric pistol squats
- Elite Beginner: Full pistol squats

Warm-Up (10-15 minutes):

- Jumping jacks: 3 minutes
- Leg swings: 10 reps each leg

- Arm circles: 10 reps each arm
- Hip circles: 10 reps each direction

Legs and Abs Workout:

- Pistol Squat Progressions:
- Body weight Squats: 2 sets x 15 reps
- Assisted Single-Leg Squats: 2 sets x 8 reps each leg
- Eccentric Pistol Squats: 3 sets x 5 reps each leg
- Full Pistol Squats (when ready): Aim for 12 reps each leg

Superset Cycles (Repeat 2x):

Cycle 1:

- Split Squats: 2 sets x 10 reps per leg
- Side lunges (Hack Squat): 2 sets x 10 reps per leg
- Lunges (Alternating Legs): 2 sets x 12 reps per leg
- Russian Twists: 2 sets x 15 reps per side

Cycle 2:

- Explosive Split Squats: 2 sets x 10 reps per leg
- Jump Squats: 2 sets x 15 reps
- L-Sit (advanced hanging L-Sit) Leg Raises: 2 sets x 10-12 reps

Finisher Exercises (Repeat 2x):

- Calf Raises: 3 sets x 15 reps
- Glute Bridges: 3 sets x 15 reps

32

Tuesday

Push Day - Advanced Upper Body Strength

Overview:

Day 2 is about advancing your upper body strength with challenging push-up variations. Continue to progress towards more advanced beginner calisthenic skills.

Progression Path:

- Beginner: Regular push-ups
- Advanced Beginner: Diamond push-ups
- Advanced: Beast pose to push-up to squat
- Elite Beginner: Tiger bend push-ups

Warm-Up (10-15 minutes):

- Jump rope: 3 minutes
- Push-up to Downward Dog: 10 reps
- Chest openers: 10 reps each side

- Wrist stretches: 1 minute

Push Day Workout:

- Regular Push-Ups: 4 sets of 12 reps
- Diamond Push-Ups: 4 sets x 10-15 reps
- Beast Pose to Push-Up to Squat: 4 sets of 10 reps
- Tiger Bend Push-Ups: Perform 4 sets of 4-12 reps (gradually increasing difficulty)
- Dips: 4 sets x 8-12 reps (band assistance if needed)
- Advanced Band overhead press: 4 sets (progress to heavier bands)
- Handstand Practice Against Wall: 4 sets x 30-60 seconds
- Pike Push-Ups: 4 sets x 8-10 reps

Finisher (Repeat 2x):

- Plank Shoulder Taps: 30 seconds
- Jumping Jacks: 30 seconds
- Mountain Climbers: 30 seconds
- Band Shoulder Press: 30 seconds
- Burpees: 5 reps

33

Wednesday

Pull Day - Advanced Upper Body and Core Strength

Overview:

Welcome to Day 3, we'll continue strengthening your upper body and core, focusing on advanced exercises that prepare you for pull-up mastery.

Progression Path:

- Beginner: Band-assisted pull-ups
- Advanced Beginner: Hanging L-sit holds
- Advanced: Band-assisted pistol squats
- Elite Beginner: Unassisted pull-ups

Warm-Up (10-15 minutes):

- Arm swings: 10 reps each arm
- Band pull-aparts: 15 reps
- Scapular shrugs: 10 reps

- Jumping jacks: 30 seconds

Pull Day Workout:

Superset Cycles (Repeat 2x):

Cycle 1:

- Band Assisted Pull-Ups: 3 sets x 6-10 reps
- Hanging L-Sit Holds: 3 sets (for time or max effort)
- Band or Chair Assisted Pistol Squats: 3 sets x 3 reps each leg

Cycle 2:

- Band Assisted Pull-Ups: 3 sets x 6-10 reps
- Hanging Knees to Elbows: 3 sets (1-10 reps, progressions)
- Band or Chair Assisted Pistol Squats: 3 sets x 3 reps each leg

Finisher Exercises:

- Band Assisted High Pulls: 4 sets x 8-12 reps
- Inverted Rows: 4 sets x 10-12 reps
- Scapular Pull-Ups: 4 sets x 8-10 reps
- Body weight Bicep Curls: 4 sets x 12-15 reps

34

Thursday

Active Rest Day – Recovery and Maintenance

Overview:

Welcome to Day 4, today is your active rest day. It's essential for recovery and maintenance. Use this time to rejuvenate and prepare for upcoming workouts. Proper recovery now will pay off when you're aiming for advanced beginner calisthenic skills in the future.

- Light Jog or Walk: 30 minutes
- Dynamic Stretching: 15 minutes
- Foam Rolling: 10 minutes

35

Friday

Full Body - Integrating Movements

Day 5 combines advanced movements to further strengthen your entire body and prepare you for advanced beginner calisthenic skills.

Progression Path:

- Beginner to Elite: Progression towards mastering each exercise

Warm-Up (10-15 minutes):

- High knees: 3 minutes
- Squat to stand: 10 reps
- Dynamic lunges: 10 reps each leg
- Shoulder circles: 10 reps each direction

Full Body Main Workout:

- Burpees: 4 sets x 15 reps

- Pull-Ups (Standard or Wide Grip): 4 sets x 6-8 reps
- Pistol Squat Progressions: 4 sets x 6 reps per leg
- Push-Ups (Variations): 4 sets x 10-15 reps
- L-Sit Progressions: 4 sets x 10-15 seconds

Finisher Circuit (Repeat 2x):

- Medicine Ball Slams: 30 seconds
- Kick Throughs: 30 seconds
- Mountain Climbers: 30 seconds
- Hollow Body Hold: 30 seconds
- Plank Shoulder Taps: 30 seconds

36

Saturday

Active Rest Day - Flexibility and Cardio
  Overview:

Day 6 is dedicated to active rest, focusing on flexibility and cardiovascular fitness. These elements are essential for balanced calisthenics training and future advanced beginner skills.

- Yoga or Light Stretching: 30 minutes
- Skipping Rope: 15 minutes

37

Sunday

Rest – Recovery and Reflection
  Overview:

On Day 7, it's time for complete rest. Allow your body and mind to recover fully, and reflect on the progress you've made this week. You're on your way to mastering the foundations of calisthenics!

38

Week 4: Progress Tracker

Please mark your progress for each exercise category. Aim to progress gradually from one category to the next. Consistency in training will lead to noticeable improvements.

Pull-Ups:

- [ ] 0-3
- [ ] 4-6
- [ ] 7-9
- [ ] 10+

Dips:

- [ ] 0-3
- [ ] 4-6
- [ ] 7-9
- [ ] 10+

L-Sit Hold:

- [ ] <10 seconds
- [ ] 10-20 seconds
- [ ] 21-30 seconds
- [ ] >30 seconds

Wall Handstand Push-Ups:

- [ ] 0-2
- [ ] 3-5
- [ ] 6-8
- [ ] 9+

One-Arm Push-Up Progressions:

- [ ] 0-1
- [ ] 2-3
- [ ] 4-5
- [ ] 6+

Chest to Bar Pull-Ups:

- [ ] 0-2
- [ ] 3-4
- [ ] 5-6
- [ ] 7+

39

You Did It!

This completes Week 4 of the program. Continue to push yourself, stay consistent, and monitor your progress. In the upcoming weeks, join us on the next workout series to take you closer to mastering intermediate calisthenics skills. Great job!

GLOSSARY

Advanced Band Overhead Press:

- **Equipment:** Resistance bands.
- **Execution:**
- Stand on the center of a resistance band with your feet shoulder-width apart.
- Grasp the resistance band handles or hold onto the band itself with both hands.
- Keep your elbows bent at a 90-degree angle with your palms facing forward.
- Your feet should be positioned firmly on the band, creating resistance.
- Push the resistance band overhead until your arms are fully extended.
- Lock your elbows at the top of the movement.
- Slowly lower the band back down to shoulder level.
- Complete the desired number of repetitions.
- **Purpose:** This exercise primarily targets the deltoid muscles (shoulders) and the triceps. It also engages the upper chest and upper back

for stability.

Arm Swings:

- **Equipment**: None (body weight exercise).
- **Execution**:
- Stand with your feet shoulder-width apart and your arms relaxed by your sides.
- Begin swinging your arms in a controlled motion, moving them forward and backward.
- Gradually increase the range of motion as you swing your arms.
- Engage your core muscles to maintain stability and control throughout the movement.
- Continue swinging your arms for the desired duration or number of repetitions.
- **Purpose**: Arm swings are a dynamic stretching exercise that helps improve shoulder mobility, increase blood flow to the upper body, and loosen up the muscles surrounding the shoulders and arms. This exercise is beneficial as a warm-up before engaging in more intense physical activity or as a standalone movement to relieve tension and improve flexibility in the shoulders and arms. Arm swings can also help enhance coordination and range of motion in the shoulder joints, making them a valuable addition to any workout routine or daily movement practice.

Assisted Single-Leg Squats:

- **Equipment:** None (body weight exercise). You may optionally use a support or chair for balance.
- **Execution:**

- Stand on one leg with the other leg extended forward.
- Lower your body by bending your standing knee while keeping the extended leg off the ground.
- Use a support or chair for balance if needed.
- Push through your heel to return to the starting position.
- **Purpose:** Assisted single-leg squats primarily target the quadriceps, hamstrings, and glutes while also challenging balance and stability. This exercise is excellent for improving lower body strength and functional fitness.

Band-Assisted Pull-Ups:

- **Equipment:** Pull-up bar, resistance band.
- **Execution:**
- Attach a resistance band to the pull-up bar.
- Place one foot or knee into the band to create assistance.
- Hang from the bar with an overhand grip.
- Pull your body up towards the bar by engaging your back and arm muscles.
- Lower yourself down with control.
- **Purpose:** Band-assisted pull-ups primarily target the latissimus dorsi (back), biceps, and shoulder muscles. This exercise serves as an effective progression towards unassisted pull-ups, helping you build strength and technique.

Band or Chair Assisted Pistol Squats:

- **Equipment:** Resistance band or chair.
- **Execution:**
- Stand on one leg with the resistance band under your other foot or use a chair for support.

- Lower your body into a pistol squat by bending your knee and hip.
- Use the band or chair for balance and assistance.
- Push through your heel to return to the starting position.
- **Purpose:** Band or chair-assisted pistol squats work the quadriceps, hamstrings, glutes, and calves. This exercise helps you develop strength, balance, and proper form for unassisted pistol squats.

Band Assisted High Pulls:

- **Equipment:** Resistance band.
- **Execution:**
- Stand on the center of a resistance band with your feet shoulder-width apart.
- Grasp the band handles or hold onto the band itself with both hands.
- Bend your knees slightly and hinge at your hips to create tension in the band.
- Pull the band towards your chest by driving your elbows upward and backward.
- Squeeze your shoulder blades together at the top of the movement.
- Lower the band back down with control.
- **Purpose:** Band-assisted high pulls target the upper back, traps, rear deltoids, and biceps. This exercise is beneficial for improving posture, strengthening the upper body, and enhancing shoulder stability.

Band-Assisted Pistol Squats:

- **Equipment:** Resistance band.
- **Execution:**
- Stand on one leg with the resistance band under your other foot.
- Hold the ends of the resistance band in each hand for stability.

- Extend your arms in front of you for balance.
- Lower your body into a squat by bending your knee and hip, keeping your torso upright.
- Use the band for support and assistance as needed to maintain balance and control.
- Keep your non-working leg extended in front of you throughout the movement.
- Push through your heel to return to the starting position.
- **Purpose**: Band-assisted pistol squats are a progression towards performing the full pistol squat exercise. They primarily target the quadriceps, hamstrings, glutes, and calves while also challenging balance and stability. By using a resistance band for support, individuals can gradually build strength and mobility in the lower body while mastering proper squatting technique. This exercise helps improve lower body strength, balance, and functional movement patterns, making it beneficial for athletes, fitness enthusiasts, and individuals seeking to enhance their overall physical performance. Incorporating band-assisted pistol squats into a workout routine can contribute to greater lower body strength, mobility, and injury prevention.

Band-Assisted Pull-Ups:

- **Equipment**: Pull-up bar, resistance band.
- **Execution**:
- Attach a resistance band to the pull-up bar, ensuring it is securely fastened.
- Step or place one foot into the bottom of the resistance band to create assistance.
- Grip the pull-up bar with your hands slightly wider than shoulder-width apart, palms facing away from you.

- Hang from the bar with your arms fully extended, engaging your core muscles.
- Pull your body up towards the bar by bending your elbows and engaging your back and arm muscles.
- Aim to bring your chin above the bar while maintaining control and proper form.
- Lower yourself down with control until your arms are fully extended, and repeat the movement.
- **Purpose:** Band-assisted pull-ups primarily target the muscles of the back, including the latissimus dorsi, biceps, and shoulders. By providing assistance, the resistance band allows individuals to perform pull-ups with proper form and technique while gradually building strength in the muscles involved. This exercise serves as an effective progression towards unassisted pull-ups, helping individuals develop the necessary strength and coordination to perform the exercise independently. Band-assisted pull-ups are beneficial for improving upper body strength, muscle definition, and functional fitness, making them a valuable addition to any strength training or calisthenics routine.

Band Face Pulls

- **Equipment:** Resistance band attached to a sturdy object at head height.
- **Execution:**
- Grab the ends of the band with both hands, palms facing down.
- Pull the band towards your face, separating your hands as you pull.
- Your hands should go beside your head. Slowly return to the start position and repeat.
- **Purpose:** Strengthens the rear deltoids, rhomboids, and traps, improving shoulder health and posture.

Band Pull-Aparts:

- **Equipment**: Resistance band.
- **Execution**:
- Stand with your feet shoulder-width apart and hold a resistance band with both hands in front of your body, palms facing downward.
- Keep a slight bend in your elbows and maintain tension in the band throughout the exercise.
- Begin by pulling the band apart horizontally, bringing your hands out to the sides until they are in line with your shoulders.
- Squeeze your shoulder blades together at the end of the movement to maximize engagement in the upper back muscles.
- Slowly return to the starting position under control, resisting the pull of the band.
- Repeat for the desired number of repetitions.
- **Purpose**: Band pull-aparts target the muscles of the upper back, including the rear deltoids, rhomboids, and trapezius. This exercise helps improve posture, strengthen the muscles responsible for scapular retraction, and prevent shoulder injuries by promoting proper shoulder mechanics. Band pull-aparts are commonly used as a warm-up or activation exercise before upper body workouts, as well as a corrective exercise to counteract the effects of prolonged sitting and forward shoulder posture.

Beast Pose to Push-Up to Squat:

- **Equipment:** None (body weight exercise).
- **Execution:**
- Begin on your hands and knees with your wrists aligned under your shoulders and knees under your hips.
- Lift your knees slightly off the ground so you're in a tabletop

position.
- Your back should be flat and parallel to the ground.
- Keep your core engaged and maintain a neutral spine.
- **Transition from Beast Pose into a Push-Up:**
- Lower your chest toward the ground by bending your elbows while keeping your body in a straight line.
- Push back up to the Beast Pose position.
- **Transition from Push-Up to Squat:**
- From the Beast Pose position, push your hips back and upward, bringing your feet forward.
- Land in a deep squat position with your feet shoulder-width apart.
- Keep your chest up and your back straight.
- **To return to the starting position, reverse the sequence:**
- Stand up from the squat position.
- Transition back into Beast Pose by placing your hands and knees on the ground.
- Repeat the sequence as needed.
- **Purpose:** This combination exercise engages the chest, shoulders, triceps, core, legs, and glutes. It challenges coordination, strength, and mobility in a full-body workout. It's an excellent exercise for building overall body strength and agility.

Beginner Band Overhead Press:

- **Equipment**: Resistance bands.
- **Execution**:
- Stand on the center of a resistance band with your feet shoulder-width apart.
- Grasp the resistance band handles or hold onto the band itself with both hands.
- Keep your elbows bent at a 90-degree angle with your palms facing

forward.

- Your feet should be positioned firmly on the band, creating resistance.
- Push the resistance band overhead until your arms are fully extended.
- Lock your elbows at the top of the movement.
- Slowly lower the band back down to shoulder level.
- **Purpose**: The beginner band overhead press primarily targets the deltoid muscles (shoulders) and the triceps. This exercise is ideal for individuals who are new to strength training or those who want to improve shoulder strength and stability. Using resistance bands allows for adjustable resistance and helps develop proper pressing mechanics while minimizing the risk of injury. Incorporating the beginner band overhead press into your routine can enhance upper body strength and promote shoulder health.

Bent Over Rows

- **Equipment:** Broomstick or light bar.
- **Execution:**
- Stand with feet shoulder-width apart, holding the broomstick with both hands, palms facing down.
- Bend your knees slightly and hinge at your waist, keeping your back straight.
- Pull the broomstick towards your lower rib cage, then lower it back down. Repeat.
- **Purpose:** Strengthens the back, biceps, and shoulders.

Bicycle Crunches:

- Equipment: None (body weight exercise).

- Execution:
- Lie on your back with your hands behind your head, elbows pointing out to the sides.
- Lift your legs off the ground, bending them at a 90-degree angle.
- Bring your right elbow towards your left knee while simultaneously straightening your right leg.
- Twist your torso, bringing your left elbow towards your right knee while straightening your left leg.
- Continue alternating sides in a pedaling motion while engaging your core.
- Purpose: Bicycle crunches target the rectus abdominis, obliques, and hip flexors. They are effective for strengthening the core and improving abdominal definition.

Body weight Bicep Curls:

- **Equipment:** None (body weight exercise).
- **Execution:**
- Stand with your feet shoulder-width apart.
- Place your hands on your hips or clasp them behind your back.
- Flex your elbow, bringing your hand towards your shoulder.
- Squeeze your bicep at the top of the movement.
- Lower your arm back down to the starting position.
- **Purpose:** Body weight bicep curls isolate and target the biceps. This simple exercise helps you build arm strength using only your body weight, making it a convenient option for bicep training.

Body weight Squats:

- **Equipment:** None (body weight exercise).
- **Execution:**

- Stand with your feet shoulder-width apart.
- Lower your body by bending your hips and knees, keeping your back straight.
- Descend until your thighs are parallel to the ground.
- Push through your heels to return to the starting position.
- **Purpose:** Body weight squats are a fundamental lower body exercise that targets the quadriceps, hamstrings, glutes, and calves. They help improve lower body strength, endurance, and overall functional fitness.

Box Jumps

- **Equipment**: Box or sturdy elevated surface.
- **Execution**:
- Stand in front of the box with feet shoulder-width apart.
- Perform a slight squat, swing your arms, and jump onto the box with both feet landing softly.
- Stand up straight, then step back down and repeat.
- **Purpose**: Improves explosive power, leg strength, and cardiovascular fitness.

Bulgarian Split Squats

- **Equipment**: None; optional bench or sturdy chair for foot elevation.
- **Execution**:
- Stand a couple of feet in front of a bench or sturdy chair. Place your rear foot on the elevated surface.
- Keeping your torso upright, lower your body until your front thigh is almost parallel to the floor.
- Ensure your front knee stays above your front foot. Push up to the starting position through your front heel.

- Repeat for the desired number of reps before switching legs.
- **Purpose**: Targets the quadriceps, hamstrings, glutes, and calves. Improves balance and unilateral leg strength.

Burpees:

- **Equipment:** None (body weight exercise).
- **Execution:**
- Begin in a standing position.
- Drop into a squat position with your hands on the ground.
- Kick your feet back into a plank position.
- Immediately return your feet into squat position.
- Explode up from the squat, jumping into the air with your arms overhead.
- **Purpose:** Burpees are a high-intensity full-body exercise that improves cardiovascular fitness, strength, and coordination.

Calf Raises:

- **Equipment:** None (body weight exercise). You can optionally use a step or elevated surface for a deeper stretch.
- **Execution:**
- Stand with your feet hip-width apart.
- Raise your heels as high as possible, lifting your body onto your toes.
- Lower your heels back down.
- You can use a step or an elevated surface to increase the range of motion and stretch the calf muscles further.
- **Purpose:** Calf raises primarily target the calf muscles (gastrocnemius and soleus). This exercise helps strengthen the calves and improve ankle stability, which is important for various activities like running and jumping.

Chair-Assisted Pistol Squats:

- **Equipment**: Chair or sturdy elevated surface.
- **Execution**:
- Stand in front of a chair or sturdy elevated surface with your feet hip-width apart.
- Extend one leg forward and slightly elevate it off the ground.
- Begin the descent by bending your standing knee and lowering your body towards the chair, keeping your chest lifted and back straight.
- Use the chair for support by lightly touching it with your fingertips or allowing your glutes to lightly touch the surface.
- Lower yourself down until your thigh is parallel to the ground or as low as your mobility allows while maintaining balance and control.
- Push through the heel of your standing leg to return to the starting position, fully extending your leg.
- Repeat for the desired number of repetitions on one leg before switching to the other leg.
- **Purpose**: Chair-assisted pistol squats are a progression towards mastering the pistol squat, a challenging single-leg exercise that requires strength, balance, and flexibility. By using a chair for support, you can gradually build the necessary lower body strength and stability while improving mobility in the hips and ankles. This exercise primarily targets the quadriceps, hamstrings, glutes, and core muscles. It's an effective way to develop unilateral leg strength and address muscle imbalances while reducing the risk of injury during the learning process.

Chest Openers:

- **Equipment**: None (body weight exercise).
- **Execution**:

- Stand tall with your feet hip-width apart and your arms relaxed by your sides.
- Interlace your fingers behind your back, palms facing each other.
- Straighten your arms and gently lift them away from your body, feeling a stretch across your chest.
- Roll your shoulders back and down to open up the chest even more.
- Keep your spine long and your chin parallel to the ground.
- Hold the stretch for 15-30 seconds while breathing deeply.
- **Purpose:** Chest openers help counteract the effects of poor posture and sedentary lifestyles by stretching the chest muscles and shoulders. They improve posture, reduce tightness in the chest and shoulders, and alleviate discomfort associated with slouching. Additionally, chest openers can increase lung capacity and improve breathing mechanics by expanding the chest cavity. Incorporating chest openers into your routine can promote better overall posture and body alignment.

Diamond Push-Ups:

- **Equipment:** None (body weight exercise).
- **Execution:**
- Perform push-ups with your hands close together under your chest, forming a diamond shape with your thumbs and index fingers.
- **Purpose:** Diamond push-ups emphasize triceps and chest muscles.

Dips:

- **Equipment:** Parallel bars or a dip station.
- **Execution:**
- Lower your body by bending your elbows until your upper arms are parallel to the ground.

- Push back up to the starting position, working the triceps and chest.
- **Purpose:** Dips target the triceps and chest muscles while also engaging the shoulders and core.

Downward Dog:

- **Equipment**: None (body weight exercise).
- **Execution**:
- Start on your hands and knees in a tabletop position, with your wrists directly under your shoulders and your knees under your hips.
- Press into your palms and lift your hips towards the ceiling, straightening your arms and legs to form an inverted V shape.
- Spread your fingers wide and press them firmly into the ground.
- Keep your head between your arms, relaxing your neck and letting it hang freely.
- Press your heels down towards the ground while lengthening through your spine and engaging your core.
- Hold the pose for the desired duration, breathing deeply and evenly.
- **Purpose**: Downward dog is a yoga pose that stretches and strengthens multiple muscle groups, including the hamstrings, calves, shoulders, and upper back. It also helps improve flexibility in the spine and releases tension in the neck and shoulders. Additionally, downward dog promotes blood circulation and can provide relief from stress and fatigue.

Dynamic Lunges:

- **Equipment**: None (body weight exercise).
- **Execution**:
- Begin in a standing position with your feet together and your arms at your sides.

- Take a large step forward with your right foot, lowering your body into a lunge position.
- Both knees should be bent at 90-degree angles, with your front thigh parallel to the ground and your back knee hovering just above the floor.
- Keep your torso upright and your core engaged for stability.
- Explosively push off your right foot to return to the starting position, bringing your right foot back next to your left.
- Immediately repeat the movement on the opposite side, stepping forward with your left foot into a lunge.
- Continue alternating legs, moving dynamically and rhythmically with each repetition.
- **Purpose**: Dynamic lunges are a compound lower body exercise that targets multiple muscle groups, including the quadriceps, hamstrings, glutes, and calves. By incorporating dynamic movements, such as stepping forward into a lunge and explosively returning to the starting position, dynamic lunges help improve lower body strength, power, and coordination. Additionally, dynamic lunges enhance hip mobility and flexibility while also providing a cardiovascular challenge, making them a versatile exercise for full-body conditioning and athletic performance. Dynamic lunges can be included in warm-up routines to prepare the body for more intense physical activity or incorporated into strength and conditioning workouts to build muscular endurance and agility.

Dynamic Stretching:

- **Equipment:** None.
- **Execution:** Perform a series of dynamic stretches that involve controlled, active movements. Examples include leg swings, arm circles, hip circles, and high knees. Aim for 15 minutes of dynamic

stretching.

- **Purpose:** Dynamic stretching helps improve flexibility, mobility, and muscle activation. It's an excellent warm-up on rest days.

Eccentric Pistol Squats:

- **Equipment:** None (body weight exercise). You may optionally use a support or chair for balance.
- **Execution:**
- Begin by standing on one leg.
- Slowly lower yourself down on the same leg, keeping the other leg extended in front.
- Use a support or chair for balance if necessary.
- Focus on the eccentric (lowering) phase of the movement.
- **Purpose:** Eccentric pistol squats primarily target the quadriceps, hamstrings, and glutes. This exercise is valuable for improving control and strength during the lowering phase of the pistol squat, which can help with overall leg strength and balance.

Explosive Split Squats:

- **Equipment:** None (body weight exercise).
- **Execution:**
- Similar to split squats but add an explosive jump when returning to the starting position.
- Jump up from the split squat position and switch legs mid-air.
- Land with the opposite leg forward.
- **Purpose:** Explosive split squats are a plyometric exercise that targets the quadriceps, hamstrings, glutes, and calves. This exercise enhances lower body power, explosiveness, and agility.

Foam Rolling:

- **Equipment:** Foam roller.
- **Execution:** Use a foam roller to target various muscle groups. Roll slowly over tight or sore areas, applying pressure as needed. Spend 10 minutes or more on foam rolling.
- **Purpose:** Foam rolling helps release muscle tension, alleviate soreness, and improve mobility. It's a valuable tool for recovery and maintenance.

Full Pistol Squats:

- **Equipment:** None (body weight exercise).
- **Execution:**
- Stand on one leg with the other leg extended forward.
- Lower your body while keeping the extended leg off the ground.
- Balance throughout the movement.
- Return to the starting position.
- **Purpose:** Full pistol squats are an advanced lower body exercise that primarily targets the quadriceps, hamstrings, and glutes. They require significant leg strength, balance, and flexibility.

Glute Bridges:

- **Equipment:** None (body weight exercise).
- **Execution:**
- Lie on your back with knees bent and feet flat on the floor.
- Lift your hips off the ground, keeping your feet and shoulders on the floor.
- Squeeze your glutes at the top and lower your hips back down.
- **Purpose:** Glute bridges target the gluteal muscles (gluteus maximus)

and hamstrings. This exercise helps strengthen the glutes, improve hip stability, and alleviate lower back discomfort.

Handstand Practice Against Wall:

- **Equipment:** Wall or vertical surface.
- **Execution:**
- Perform handstands with your feet against a wall for stability and balance.
- **Purpose:** Handstand practice against a wall strengthens the shoulders, arms, and core while improving balance and helping you progress toward freestanding handstands.

Hanging Knees to Elbows:

- **Equipment:** Pull-up bar or hanging apparatus.
- **Execution:**
- Hang from the bar with your arms fully extended.
- Bend your knees and raise them toward your chest.
- Simultaneously, bring your elbows down and back, aiming to touch your knees.
- Lower your legs and repeat the movement.
- **Purpose:** Hanging knees to elbows primarily target the abdominal muscles, specifically the lower abs and obliques. It also engages the lats and shoulder stabilizers, contributing to core strength and stability.

Hanging L-Sit Holds:

- **Equipment:** Pull-up bar or parallel bars.
- **Execution:**

- Hang from the bar with your arms fully extended.
- Lift your legs up, keeping them straight, until they are parallel to the ground.
- Hold this position for the desired duration.
- **Purpose:** Hanging L-sit holds are an advanced core exercise that challenges the entire core, including the lower abs, upper abs, and hip flexors. It also improves grip strength and overall body control.

Hanging Leg Raises

- **Equipment:** Pull-up bar.
- **Execution:**
- Hang from a pull-up bar with your legs straight.
- Raise your legs in front of you while keeping them straight, until they are parallel to the ground.
- Slowly lower them back down and repeat.
- **Purpose:** Targets the core, specifically the lower abdominals, and improves grip strength.

Hollow Body Hold:

- **Equipment:** None (body weight exercise).
- **Execution:** Lie on your back with arms and legs extended. Lift your head, shoulders, arms, and legs off the ground. Maintain a hollow shape with your lower back pressed into the floor.
- **Purpose:** The hollow body hold strengthens the core and improves body awareness.

High Knees:

- **Equipment**: None (body weight exercise).

- **Execution**:
- Begin in a standing position with your feet hip-width apart and arms at your sides.
- Engage your core muscles to stabilize your torso.
- Lift your right knee towards your chest as high as possible while simultaneously driving your left arm forward.
- Lower your right leg back to the ground and immediately repeat the movement with your left leg, driving your right arm forward.
- Continue alternating legs in a running motion, moving at a quick pace to elevate your heart rate.
- Maintain a light bounce on the balls of your feet throughout the exercise.
- **Purpose**: High knees are a dynamic cardiovascular exercise that engages multiple muscle groups, including the quadriceps, hip flexors, hamstrings, and core muscles. This exercise helps improve agility, coordination, and lower body strength while also increasing heart rate and calorie burn. High knees are commonly used as a warm-up exercise before more intense workouts or as part of a high-intensity interval training (HIIT) routine to enhance cardiovascular fitness and endurance. Additionally, high knees can be incorporated into sports-specific training programs to improve running mechanics and sprinting speed.

Incline Push-Ups

- **Equipment**: Sturdy bench, step, or platform.
- **Execution**:
- Place your hands on the edge of the elevated surface, slightly wider than shoulder-width apart.
- Step your feet back so your body is in a straight line. Keeping your core tight, lower your chest to the edge of the surface and push back

up to the start position.

- **Purpose**: Targets the lower chest and shoulders, slightly easier than regular push-ups, suitable for building strength for more advanced variations.

Inverted Rows:

- **Equipment:** Horizontal bar or Smith machine.
- **Execution:**
- Lie on your back under the bar.
- Grab the bar with an overhand grip, palms facing away from you.
- Keep your body straight and heels on the ground.
- Pull your chest towards the bar by bending your elbows.
- Lower your body back down with control.
- **Purpose:** Inverted rows target the upper back, lats, rear deltoids, and biceps. This body weight exercise is effective for developing upper body strength and improving posture.

Jump Squats:

- **Equipment:** None (body weight exercise).
- **Execution:**
- Begin in a squat position.
- Explosively jump up and extend your legs fully.
- Land softly and return to the squat position.
- **Purpose:** Jump squats are a plyometric exercise that enhances lower body power, explosiveness, and overall leg strength. They also provide a cardiovascular benefit.

Jumping Jacks:

- **Equipment:** None (body weight exercise).
- **Execution:**
- Begin in a standing position with arms at your sides.
- Simultaneously jump your legs outward and raise your arms above your head.
- Return to the starting position by jumping your legs together and lowering your arms.
- **Purpose:** Jumping jacks provide a cardiovascular workout, improve coordination, and serve as an effective warm-up exercise.

Jumping Lunges:

- **Equipment**: None (body weight exercise).
- **Execution**:
- Start in a lunge position with one leg forward and one leg back.
- Lower your body into a lunge, ensuring both knees are bent at 90-degree angles.
- Explosively jump into the air, switching the position of your legs mid-air.
- Land softly with the opposite leg forward and immediately lower into another lunge.
- Continue alternating legs for the desired number of repetitions.
- **Purpose**: Jumping lunges are a plyometric exercise that targets the quadriceps, hamstrings, glutes, and calves. They improve lower body strength, power, and explosiveness.

Jumping Lunges:

- Equipment: None (body weight exercise).
- Execution:
- Start in a lunge position with one leg forward and one leg back.

- Lower your body into a lunge, ensuring both knees are bent at 90-degree angles.
- Explosively jump into the air, switching the position of your legs mid-air.
- Land softly with the opposite leg forward and immediately lower into another lunge.
- Continue alternating legs for the desired number of repetitions.
- Purpose: Jumping lunges are a plyometric exercise that targets the quadriceps, hamstrings, glutes, and calves. They improve lower body strength, power, and explosiveness.

Jumping Pull-Ups

- **Equipment:** Pull-up bar.
- **Execution:**
- Stand under a pull-up bar.
- Jump and pull yourself up simultaneously so that your chin reaches above the bar.
- Let yourself down slowly after the jump. Repeat.
- **Purpose:** Helps build strength and technique for full pull-ups, engaging the upper body muscles.

Kick Throughs:

- **Equipment**: None (body weight exercise).
- **Execution**:
- Start in a push-up position with your hands placed directly under your shoulders and your body forming a straight line from head to heels.
- Lift your right hand off the ground and rotate your body to the left, simultaneously kicking your right leg through the space under your

body.

- Extend your right leg fully and rotate your hips to face upward as you bring your leg across your body.
- Your left hand and foot should support your body weight as you pivot on your toes.
- Reverse the movement by bringing your right leg back to the starting position and returning your right hand to the ground.
- Repeat the motion on the opposite side, kicking your left leg through and rotating your body to the right.
- Continue alternating sides in a fluid and controlled manner.
- **Purpose**: Kick throughs are a dynamic body weight exercise that targets the core, shoulders, and hip flexors while also improving agility and coordination. This exercise helps to strengthen the muscles of the core and upper body while enhancing rotational stability and mobility. By incorporating both upper and lower body movements in a coordinated manner, kick throughs promote functional strength and athleticism. Additionally, the dynamic nature of the exercise provides a cardiovascular challenge, making it an effective addition to high-intensity interval training (HIIT) workouts or circuit training routines. Including kick throughs in your workout regimen can help enhance overall fitness, agility, and body control.

Leg Raises

- **Equipment**: None; mat optional for comfort.
- **Execution**:
- Lie flat on your back with your legs straight and hands beneath your lower back for support.
- Keeping your legs straight, lift them up to the ceiling until your butt comes slightly off the floor. Slowly lower them back down just above

the floor.

- Repeat for the desired number of reps.
- **Purpose**: Strengthens the lower abdominals and hip flexors.

Lunges (Alternating Legs):

- **Equipment:** None (body weight exercise).
- **Execution:**
- Stand with your feet hip-width apart.
- Take a step forward and lower your body until both knees are bent at a 90-degree angle.
- Push off the front foot to return to the starting position.
- Alternate legs.
- **Purpose:** Lunges primarily target the quadriceps, hamstrings, and glutes while also engaging the calves and core muscles. They improve lower body strength and balance.

L-Sit (Advanced Hanging L-Sit) Leg Raises:

- **Equipment:** Hang from a pull-up bar or parallel bars.
- **Execution:**
- Lift your legs up, keeping them straight, until they are parallel to the ground.
- Hold this position.
- **Purpose:** L-Sit leg raises target the abdominal muscles, hip flexors, and shoulder stabilizers. This exercise improves core strength, hip flexor flexibility, and overall stability.

L-Sit (on the Floor) Leg Raises

- **Equipment**: None.

- **Execution**:
- Sit on the floor with your legs straight ahead and your hands placed beside your hips.
- Press down into the floor with your hands to lift your body slightly. Keeping your legs straight, raise them as high as possible.
- Lower them back down without touching the floor.
- Repeat for reps.
- **Purpose**: Primarily targets the core muscles, improving strength and stability, with additional engagement of the hip flexors.

L-Sit Progressions:

- **Equipment:** Parallel bars or parallettes.
- **Execution:** Start with L-sit progressions, which involve lifting your legs while seated on parallel bars.
- **Purpose:** L-sit progressions build core strength, hip flexor flexibility, and stability.

Light Jog or Walk:

- **Equipment:** None.
- **Execution:** Go for a light jog or brisk walk at a comfortable pace. Duration may vary based on your fitness level, but aim for around 30 minutes.
- **Purpose:** Light jogging or walking on rest days helps improve blood circulation, aids in recovery, and maintains overall cardiovascular health.

Medicine Ball Chest Pass

- **Equipment**: Medicine ball.

- **Execution:**
- Stand facing a sturdy wall about a couple of feet away, holding a medicine ball at chest level.
- Explosively push the ball away from your chest to throw it against the wall, then catch it on the rebound.
- Repeat for the desired number of reps.
- **Purpose:** Develops explosive upper body power, strengthens chest, shoulders, and triceps.

Medicine Ball Slams:

- **Equipment**: Medicine ball.
- **Execution**:
- Stand with your feet shoulder-width apart, holding a medicine ball overhead.
- Engage your core muscles and maintain a slight bend in your knees.
- With explosive force, slam the medicine ball onto the ground directly in front of you.
- As you slam the ball, bend forward at the waist and hinge your hips to generate power.
- Keep your arms extended throughout the movement, using your entire body to drive the ball downward.
- Catch the ball on the bounce or as it rebounds off the ground.
- Immediately repeat the movement for the desired number of repetitions.
- **Purpose**: Medicine ball slams are a dynamic and high-intensity exercise that targets multiple muscle groups, including the core, shoulders, arms, and legs. By incorporating explosive movements and full-body coordination, this exercise helps to develop power, strength, and cardiovascular fitness. Medicine ball slams also provide an effective outlet for releasing tension and stress, making

them a popular choice for both athletic training and general fitness. Additionally, the rhythmic and repetitive nature of the exercise can help improve coordination, agility, and mental focus. Including medicine ball slams in your workout routine can add variety and challenge while promoting functional strength and athleticism.

Mountain Climbers:

- **Equipment**: None (body weight exercise).
- **Execution**:
- Begin in a plank position with your hands directly under your shoulders and your body forming a straight line from head to heels.
- Engage your core and keep your hips stable as you lift your right foot off the ground and bring your right knee towards your chest.
- Quickly switch legs by extending your right leg back to the starting position while simultaneously bringing your left knee towards your chest.
- Continue alternating legs in a running motion, moving at a rapid pace while maintaining proper form.
- Aim to keep your shoulders, hips, and feet aligned throughout the exercise, avoiding any excessive bouncing or sagging in the lower back.
- **Purpose**: Mountain climbers are a dynamic full-body exercise that targets multiple muscle groups, including the core, shoulders, chest, and legs. This exercise helps to improve cardiovascular endurance, agility, and coordination while also strengthening the muscles of the core and upper body. Mountain climbers are particularly effective for building core stability and strength, as they require the engagement of abdominal and lower back muscles to maintain proper form throughout the movement. Additionally, the rapid alternating motion of the legs elevates the heart rate, making mountain climbers

an excellent choice for cardiovascular conditioning and calorie burning. Incorporating mountain climbers into your workouts can help enhance overall fitness levels and contribute to a stronger, more resilient body.

Negative Pull-Ups

- **Equipment:** Pull-up bar.
- **Execution:**
- Jump or use a step to get your chin above the bar with an overhand grip.
- Slowly lower yourself with a controlled motion until your arms are fully extended.
- Step back onto the platform and repeat.
- **Purpose:** Builds strength in the back, biceps, and grip, especially focusing on the eccentric (lowering) phase of the pull-up.

Pike Push-Ups:

- **Equipment:** None (body weight exercise).
- **Execution:**
- Begin in a downward dog yoga pose with your hands shoulder-width apart and your hips lifted high towards the ceiling.
- Walk your feet towards your hands, bringing your body into an inverted "V" shape with your hips raised and legs straight.
- Ensure that your head is positioned between your arms, and your gaze is towards your feet.
- Lower your upper body towards the ground by bending your elbows, allowing your head to move towards the floor.
- Keep your elbows close to your body as you lower yourself down.
- Push through your palms to extend your arms and return to the

starting position, maintaining the pike position throughout the movement.

- **Purpose**: Pike push-ups target the shoulders, triceps, and chest muscles while also engaging the core and improving shoulder mobility. This exercise is particularly effective for building shoulder strength and stability, as it requires the deltoids and triceps to support the body weight in an inverted position. Pike push-ups are a beneficial progression towards handstand push-ups and can help individuals develop the necessary strength and technique for more advanced shoulder exercises. Additionally, the pike position places greater emphasis on the anterior deltoids, making it a valuable exercise for developing well-rounded shoulder strength and definition. Incorporating pike push-ups into your workout routine can help you build upper body strength, improve shoulder stability, and enhance overall athletic performance.

Pistol Squats:

- **Equipment**: None (body weight exercise).
- **Execution**:
- Begin by standing on one leg with the other leg extended forward.
- Lower your body while keeping the extended leg off the ground, maintaining balance and control.
- Descend into a squat position by bending your standing knee and hip, keeping your back straight and chest lifted.
- Lower yourself down as far as your mobility allows, aiming to bring your thigh parallel to the ground or lower.
- Keep your heel firmly planted on the ground and your knee aligned with your toes throughout the movement.
- Push through the heel of your standing leg to return to the starting position, fully extending your leg.

- Repeat for the desired number of repetitions on one leg before switching to the other leg.
- **Purpose**: Pistol squats are an advanced body weight exercise that targets the quadriceps, hamstrings, glutes, and core muscles. They require significant lower body strength, balance, and flexibility. By performing pistol squats, you can improve unilateral leg strength, address muscle imbalances, and enhance overall lower body functional fitness. Additionally, pistol squats challenge proprioception and stability, making them beneficial for athletes and individuals seeking to improve athletic performance and injury resilience.

Plank:

- **Equipment**: None (body weight exercise).
- **Execution**:
- Start in a push-up position with your hands directly under your shoulders and your body forming a straight line from head to heels.
- Engage your core muscles and hold this position, keeping your abs and glutes tight.
- Avoid sagging your hips or lifting your buttocks too high.
- Focus on maintaining a neutral spine and breathing rhythmically.
- Hold the plank for the desired duration.
- **Purpose**: Planks are a static core exercise that targets the entire core, including the rectus abdominis, transverse abdominis, obliques, and lower back muscles. They improve core strength, stability, and endurance.

Plank Shoulder Taps:

- **Equipment:** None (body weight exercise).
- **Execution:**

- Start in a plank position on your hands.
- Lift one hand off the ground and touch your opposite shoulder.
- Alternate sides while maintaining a stable core.
- **Purpose:** Plank shoulder taps challenge core stability and shoulder strength while promoting balance and coordination.

Pull-Ups (Standard or Wide Grip):

- **Equipment:** Pull-up bar.
- **Execution:** Hang from the bar with your hands in a standard or wide grip. Pull your body up towards the bar until your chin clears it. Lower your body back down with control.
- **Purpose:** Pull-ups target the back, biceps, and shoulders, enhancing upper body strength and muscle development.

Push-Ups (Variations):

- **Equipment:** None (body weight exercise).
- **Execution:** Perform push-ups with various hand placements, such as wide, close, or diamond. Maintain proper form, keeping your body in a straight line.
- **Purpose:** Push-ups strengthen the chest, shoulders, triceps, and core. Variations target different muscle groups.

Regular Push-Ups:

- **Equipment:** None (body weight exercise).
- **Execution:**
- Begin in a plank position with your hands shoulder-width apart.
- Lower your body by bending your elbows.
- Push back up to the starting position, targeting chest, triceps, and

shoulders.

- **Purpose:** Regular push-ups strengthen the chest, shoulders, triceps, and core. They are a fundamental body weight exercise for upper body strength.

Russian Twists:

- **Equipment:** None (body weight exercise). You may optionally use a weight or object for resistance.
- **Execution:**
- Sit on the floor with your knees bent, heels on the ground, and back at a slight angle.
- Hold a weight or object with both hands.
- Twist your torso to one side, bringing the object close to the floor.
- Return to the center and twist to the other side.
- **Purpose:** Russian twists primarily target the obliques and core muscles. They improve core strength, rotational stability, and spinal mobility.

Shoulder Circles:

- **Equipment**: None (body weight exercise).
- **Execution**:
- Stand with your feet shoulder-width apart and your arms hanging naturally at your sides.
- Begin by gently rolling your shoulders forward in a circular motion.
- As you complete the forward circle, gradually increase the size of the movement, allowing your shoulders to move freely.
- After several repetitions, reverse the motion and roll your shoulders backward in a circular motion.
- Again, gradually increase the size of the circles as you continue the

movement.

- Maintain smooth and controlled movements throughout the exercise, avoiding any sudden or jerky motions.
- **Purpose**: Shoulder circles are a simple yet effective exercise for improving shoulder mobility, flexibility, and range of motion. By performing circular movements with the shoulders, this exercise helps to loosen up tight muscles, reduce stiffness, and alleviate tension in the shoulder joint. Shoulder circles can be particularly beneficial for individuals who spend long periods sitting or working at a desk, as they help counteract the forward-leaning posture commonly associated with sedentary lifestyles. Additionally, shoulder circles are a valuable warm-up exercise before engaging in more strenuous activities, such as weightlifting or overhead movements, as they help prepare the shoulders for increased intensity and reduce the risk of injury. Incorporating shoulder circles into your regular exercise routine can contribute to overall shoulder health and function, promoting better posture and movement patterns.

Side Lunges (Hack Squat):

- **Equipment:** None (body weight exercise).
- **Execution:**
- Take a wide step to the side.
- Bend one knee while keeping the other leg straight.
- Push your hips back and return to the starting position.
- Alternate sides.
- **Purpose:** Side lunges, also known as hack squats, target the quadriceps, hamstrings, adductors, and glutes. They enhance leg strength, flexibility, and lateral movement.

Split Squats:

- **Equipment:** None (body weight exercise).
- **Execution:**
- Stand with one foot forward and the other foot extended behind you.
- Lower your body by bending both knees.
- Return to the starting position.
- Repeat on the other leg.
- **Purpose:** Split squats primarily target the quadriceps, hamstrings, glutes, and calves. This exercise improves lower body strength, balance, and single-leg stability.

Scapular Pull-Ups:

- **Equipment:** Pull-up bar.
- **Execution:**
- Hang from the bar with your arms fully extended.
- Keep your arms straight and pull your shoulder blades down and together.
- Hold this position for a moment.
- Relax your shoulder blades and return to the starting position.
- **Purpose:** Scapular pull-ups focus on the scapular muscles and shoulder stability. They help improve scapular mobility and posture while enhancing shoulder health and function.

Scapular Shrugs:

- **Equipment:** None (body weight exercise).
- **Execution:**
- Stand with your feet shoulder-width apart and arms relaxed by your sides.
- Focus on your shoulder blades (scapulae). Without moving your arms, raise and squeeze your shoulder blades together as if you're

trying to touch them behind your back.

- Hold this position for a moment to emphasize the contraction of the scapular muscles.
- Relax and return to the starting position.
- **Purpose:** Scapular shrugs help improve scapular mobility and stability. They activate and strengthen the muscles responsible for proper shoulder blade movement, which is essential for overall shoulder health and posture.

Standing Wall Angels:

- **Equipment:** Wall or vertical surface.
- **Execution:** Stand with your back against a wall or vertical surface. Place your feet about hip-width apart and ensure your entire spine, from head to lower back, is in contact with the wall. Bend your elbows to 90-degree angles with your arms out to the sides, resembling a "goalpost" position. Slowly slide your arms upward along the wall, maintaining contact with your elbows and wrists. Once your arms are fully extended overhead, slowly lower them back down to the starting position.
- **Purpose:** Standing wall angels are an excellent exercise for improving shoulder mobility, posture, and upper body flexibility. They help activate and strengthen the muscles responsible for maintaining proper posture while promoting a wider range of motion in the shoulder joints. This exercise is particularly beneficial for those who spend long hours sitting or working at a computer.

Superman Planks:

- **Equipment**: None (body weight exercise).
- **Execution**:

- Start in a plank position with your forearms on the ground and your body in a straight line from head to heels.
- Engage your core and lift one arm and the opposite leg off the ground simultaneously, reaching them out in front of you and behind you, respectively.
- Hold this extended position for a moment, keeping your body stable and parallel to the ground.
- Lower your arm and leg back to the starting position and repeat on the opposite side.
- **Purpose**: Superman planks target the muscles of the core, lower back, glutes, and shoulders. This exercise improves core strength, stability, and endurance while also helping to enhance posture and spinal alignment. By engaging multiple muscle groups simultaneously, superman planks promote functional strength and overall athleticism. Incorporating superman planks into your workout routine can contribute to improved core stability and injury prevention while supporting optimal performance in various activities and sports.

Tiger Bend Push-Ups:

- **Equipment:** None (body weight exercise).
- **Execution:**
- Perform push-ups while tucking your elbows close to your body and bending at the waist.
- **Purpose:** Tiger bend push-ups emphasize triceps and shoulder strength.

Tricep Dips:

- **Equipment**: Parallel bars or a dip station.
- **Execution**:
- Position yourself between the parallel bars or on the dip station with your hands gripping the bars and arms fully extended.
- Keep your elbows close to your body as you lower your body by bending your elbows until your upper arms are parallel to the ground or slightly below.
- Push back up to the starting position, straightening your arms and engaging your triceps.
- **Purpose**: Tricep dips primarily target the triceps muscles, with secondary involvement of the chest, shoulders, and core muscles. This exercise is effective for strengthening the triceps and improving upper body pushing strength. Tricep dips can be performed with body weight or additional resistance to progressively overload the triceps muscles for greater strength and muscle development. Incorporating tricep dips into your workout routine can help you build strong and defined arms while enhancing overall upper body strength and muscular endurance.

Unassisted Pull-Ups:

- **Equipment**: Pull-up bar.
- **Execution**:
- Grip the pull-up bar with your hands slightly wider than shoulder-width apart, palms facing away from you.
- Hang from the bar with your arms fully extended.
- Engage your core and pull yourself up towards the bar by bending your elbows and pulling your shoulder blades down and back.
- Continue pulling until your chin clears the bar.
- Lower yourself back down with control until your arms are fully extended.

- Repeat for the desired number of repetitions.
- **Purpose**: Unassisted pull-ups are a challenging body weight exercise that primarily target the latissimus dorsi (back), biceps, and shoulder muscles. They are an excellent measure of upper body strength and can help improve overall functional fitness. Incorporating unassisted pull-ups into a workout routine can enhance back and arm strength, improve grip strength, and contribute to a well-rounded upper body development. Progressing to unassisted pull-ups from assisted variations signifies significant strength gains and mastery of body weight movements. By consistently practicing unassisted pull-ups, individuals can build muscle mass, increase upper body strength, and achieve their fitness goals.

Wide Push-Ups

- **Equipment**: None.
- **Execution**:
- Begin in a push-up position with your hands set wider than shoulder-width apart.
- Lower your body to the floor, keeping elbows slightly tucked in.
- Push back up to the starting position.
- **Purpose**: Targets the chest, with an emphasis on the outer chest muscles, as well as the shoulders and triceps.

Yoga or Light Stretching:

- **Equipment:** Yoga mat or comfortable surface.
- **Execution:** Engage in a yoga session or perform light stretching exercises. Focus on improving flexibility, balance, and relaxation. Allocate around 30 minutes for yoga or stretching.
- **Purpose:** Yoga and stretching routines enhance flexibility, reduce

muscle tension, and promote mental well-being.